# YOUR KNOWLEDGE HAS VALUE

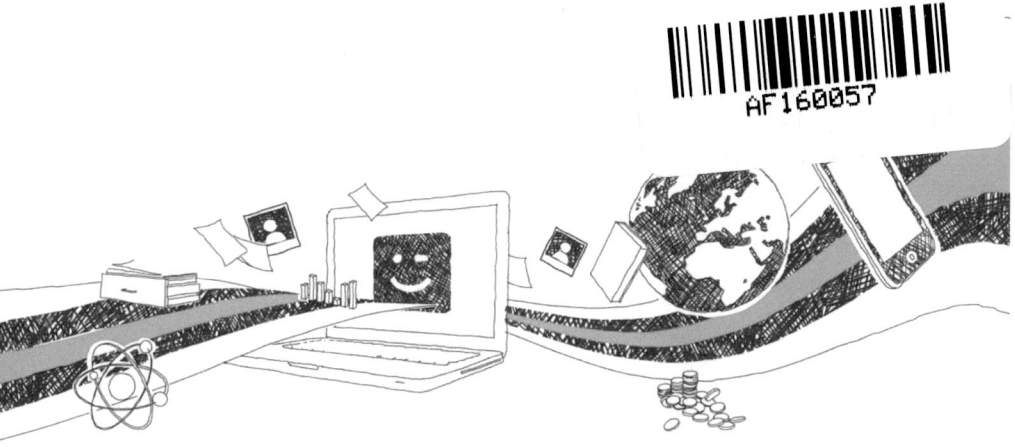

- We will publish your bachelor's and master's thesis, essays and papers

- Your own eBook and book - sold worldwide in all relevant shops

- Earn money with each sale

Upload your text at www.GRIN.com
and publish for free

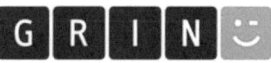

**Bibliographic information published by the German National Library:**

The German National Library lists this publication in the National Bibliography; detailed bibliographic data are available on the Internet at http://dnb.dnb.de .

This book is copyright material and must not be copied, reproduced, transferred, distributed, leased, licensed or publicly performed or used in any way except as specifically permitted in writing by the publishers, as allowed under the terms and conditions under which it was purchased or as strictly permitted by applicable copyright law. Any unauthorized distribution or use of this text may be a direct infringement of the author s and publisher s rights and those responsible may be liable in law accordingly.

**Imprint:**

Copyright © 2018 GRIN Verlag, Open Publishing GmbH
Print and binding: Books on Demand GmbH, Norderstedt Germany
ISBN: 9783668624191

**This book at GRIN:**

https://www.grin.com/document/388414

Patrick Kimuyu

# Pathophysiology of Acontractile Smooth Muscle Syndrome

GRIN Publishing

**GRIN - Your knowledge has value**

Since its foundation in 1998, GRIN has specialized in publishing academic texts by students, college teachers and other academics as e-book and printed book. The website www.grin.com is an ideal platform for presenting term papers, final papers, scientific essays, dissertations and specialist books.

**Visit us on the internet:**

http://www.grin.com/

http://www.facebook.com/grincom

http://www.twitter.com/grin_com

# Content

Introduction .................................................................................................................. 2

Mechanism of Smooth Muscles ................................................................................... 2

Organs with Smooth Muscles ...................................................................................... 5

Possible Causes of Symptoms Associated with ASMS ................................................. 6

Conclusion .................................................................................................................... 8

References ................................................................................................................... 9

## Introduction

Due to extensive epidemiological studies and technological advancements in the field of medicine, new diseases are being regularly discovered. Understanding human physiology and pathophysiology has enhanced the search for cures and therapeutic remedies to most diseases. However, some health conditions are accompanied by unprecedented controversy owing to the absence of known etiological causes. In most cases, knowing the aetiology of a certain disease helps in developing medicines and treatment therapies, in order to cure the disease or manage the disease symptoms, as it is the case with chronic illnesses. In this case study, the pathophysiology of Acontractile Smooth Muscle Syndrome (ASMS) seems easy to understand because its cause is known. The fact that ASMS is caused by a genetic mutation of recessive genes implies that it affects tissues and organs which have smooth muscles (Webb, 2003). Therefore, this paper will present a number of hypotheses on the possible pathophysiology of ASMS.

## Mechanism of Smooth Muscles

It is arguable that ASMS causes changes in smooth muscle physiology in the affected body tissue and organs. As such, the mechanism of smooth muscles in the affected organs is impaired and this is manifested by the characteristic symptoms which are associated with the smooth muscle disorder. ASMS is characterised by lymphedema, cyanosis and increased incidence of urinary tract infections. In addition, it is reported that ASMS causes systolic heart failure, the leading cause of death in people with the disorder although ASMS is not known to have a direct effect on the contractility of cardiac muscles. However, the pathophysiology of ASMS is not known.

ASMS is reported to have reduced ability of smooth muscle to either relax or contract, leaving it rigid or acontractile. Therefore, it is apparent that this disorder disrupts the physiology of smooth muscles in the body. As such, it is worth discerning the general mechanism of smooth muscles, although different types of smooth muscles in different organs exhibit differences in their functioning. These changes are attributable to the differences in the activation of the respective muscle cells. Nevertheless, the outcome of muscle cell activation leads to the contraction and relaxation of all smooth muscles regardless of their types and location in the body (Webb, 2003).

In the body, the contractile mechanism of smooth muscles involves the mechanical activation of myosin and actin which are the principal contractile proteins. In most cases, contraction of the smooth muscles is triggered by the activation of stretch-dependent $Ca^{2+}$ channels which are located on the plasma membrane owing to changes in membrane potential. During smooth muscle contraction, contractile proteins, myosin and actin, interact under the influence of myosin light chain (MLC) kinase which controls the phosphorylation of myosin end plates. On the other hand, ATPase is involved in the process of energy generation for the binding of myosin and actin proteins. This enzyme catalyses the release of ATP energy which is utilised in the binding of myosin and actin. This results in a contraction due to the cycling of myosin cross-bridges with actin end-plates. Therefore, it is worth noting that contractility of smooth muscles is a highly regulated process which is determined by the activity of myosin light chain kinase and ATPase (Webb, 2003).

In smooth muscle contractions, changes in calcium ions across the plasma membrane control the contractile activity of smooth muscles. Ordinarily, $Ca^{2+}$-mediated changes in the thick filaments are responsible for contraction. This phenomenon is different from the one occurring in striated muscles in skeletal tissues in which $Ca^{2+}$-mediated changes in the thin filaments causes muscle contractility. Calcium ion-dependent contraction of smooth muscles is triggered by specific stimuli which cause an increase in calcium ions in the intracellular space of the smooth muscle cell. As a result, the acid protein, calmodulin, combines with calcium ions to form an activator complex. In turn, the complex formed by the combination of calcium ions and calmodulin activates myosin light chain kinase which is responsible for phosphorylating the light chain of myosin. On the other hand, the increase of cytosolic $Ca^{2+}$ which is caused by the release of $Ca^{2+}$ from the sarcoplasmic reticulum, an intracellular store for calcium, and entry of $Ca^{2+}$ from the extracellular space through receptor-operated $Ca^{2+}$ channels, leads to the stimulation of phospholipase C activity. This enzyme catalyses the formation of diacylglycerol (DG) and inositol triphosphate (IP3) from a lipid known as phosphatidylinositol 4, 5-bisphosphate, a principal membrane lipid. These two compounds act as messengers in which IP3 triggers the release of $Ca^{2+}$ by the sarcoplasmic reticulum, whereas diacylglycerol activates protein kinase C under the influence of high $Ca^{2+}$ concentration. As a result, protein kinase C phosphorylates the light chain of myosin; thus, causing cross-bridge cycling (Webb, 2003).

Smooth muscles in lymphatic, airway and vascular system have an endogenous pacemaker mechanism which is controlled by a cytosolic $Ca^{2+}$ oscillator to generate rhythmical contractions which are known to last for an extended period (Berridge, 2008). However, the mechanism of contraction is the same in all smooth muscles despite the differences involved in the activation process.

The second phase of smooth muscle activity is the relaxation phase which occurs after contraction. As such, relaxation of the smooth muscles occurs after the removal of the contractile stimuli. Therefore, this phase occurs at low cytosolic $Ca^{2+}$ concentration coupled to the increased activity of myosin light chain phosphatase which is responsible for the dephosphorylation of myosin cross-bridges. Evidence shows that the relaxation of smooth muscles is caused by a decrease in the intracellular concentration of $Ca^{2+}$ and this occurs through a number of physiological mechanisms. First, $Ca^{2+}$-binding proteins in smooth muscles such as calreticulin and calsequestrin prevent the release of Ca2+ from the sarcoplasmic reticulum which leads to decreased intracellular $Ca^{2+}$ concentration. Second, the entry of $Ca^{2+}$ from the extracellular space is blocked by the activity of Ca/Mg-ATPases which stimulate plasma membrane $Ca^{2+}$ pump by binding with calmodulin. As a result, the stimulated plasma membrane $Ca^{2+}$ pumps calcium ions from the cytosolic space of smooth muscle cells leading to a decrease in intracellular $Ca^{2+}$ concentration. This process is enhanced by the activity of $Na+/Ca^{2+}$ exchangers located on the plasma membrane (Berridge, 2008).

During the relaxation of smooth muscles, myosin light chain cross-bridges with actin breaks up because of the effect of phosphorylation of myosin light chain by myosin light chain phosphatase. As a result, the contractile smooth muscle returns to a relaxed state.

## Organs with Smooth Muscles

In the body, smooth muscles are found in different tissues and organs. Reproductive systems, especially the uterus and vas deferens, have smooth muscle cells which play different roles. In vas deferens, smooth muscles are responsible for the rapid peristaltic contractions during ejaculation of the sperms. On the other hand, smooth muscles in the uterus are responsible for the weak twitches experienced during early pregnancy and the onset of labour. Smooth muscles are also found in the bladder and the ureter. The ureter smooth muscles aid in the transfer of urine from the kidney to the bladder and the urethral smooth muscles are responsible for the passage of urine. The bladder is also surrounded by layers of destrusor smooth muscle cells which are involved in the bladder contractions during the expulsion of urine. It is also worth noting that smooth muscles are found in the gastrointestinal tract, airways, lymphatic and the vascular system where they generate rhythmic contractions (Berridge, 2008).Therefore, this suggests that ASMS affects some, possibly all, of these organs and tissues which rely on smooth muscles for different functions.

In most cases, alterations in the mechanism of smooth muscles, especially in the phosphorylation of the myosin light chain proteins and the maintenance of intracellular $Ca^{2+}$, have been found to be responsible for the abnormal contractile activities in smooth muscles cells of the affected organs and tissues. In addition, alterations by genetic defects in the upstream targets which cause impacts on myosin light chain phosphorylation and $Ca^{2+}$ levels have also been found to cause abnormal smooth muscle contractile events in some organs. Therefore, it is possible that ASMS causes similar alterations in smooth muscles which impair the contraction and relaxation mechanism of smooth muscle cells in the affected organs and tissues.

## Possible Causes of Symptoms Associated with ASMS

It appears that ASMS affects the smooth muscles in the lymphatic, vascular and the respiratory systems. This assertion can be justified by the pathophysiology involved in producing the main symptoms. ASMS is said to be characterised by lymphedema, cyanosis and increased urinary tract infections. In addition, the effects of ASMS are reported to be associated with the left systolic heart failure in most patients, especially in newborns.

Cyanosis is defined as the bluish discoloration of the mucus membrane, skin and nail beds. Clinically, cyanosis has been found to occur when deoxygenated haemoglobin in the blood circulation reaches 5gm/dl (Martin, 2013). At such levels, blood appears bluish or purple, and this explains why mucus membranes and skin turn bluish in their appearance. In practice, cyanosis is caused by a number of factors including severe problems with circulation, breathing and airway, especially in newborns. This is referred to as central cyanosis. Another form of cyanosis, referred to as peripheral cyanosis, occurs commonly in adults and it is caused by reduced cardiac output and constriction of blood vessels especially in the limbs, toes and fingers. Therefore, the occurrence of cyanosis in ASMS suggests an abnormality in airway smooth muscles which leads to impaired breathing. As a result, the uptake of oxygen by haemoglobin is compromised and this explains why deoxygenated haemoglobin levels rise beyond 5 gm/dl, the level upon which cyanosis is manifested through the bluish discoloration of the mucus membranes and skin. ASMS may also be causing cyanosis through causing constriction of blood capillaries.

Lymphedema refers to a chronic swelling which is caused by the failure of lymphatic drainage leading to the accumulation of lymph fluid in the tissues. This condition is usually observed in the extremities such as the legs and arms. Evidence shows that lymphedema results from the blockage of the lymphatic vessels. Therefore, the occurrence of lymphedema as one of the main symptoms of ASMS suggests that this disorder affects the lymphatic smooth muscle cells. The lymphatic system fails to drain lymph fluid from the tissues, a phenomenon which is manifested through swelling of the extremities. It is reported that developmental abnormalities of the lymphatic system causes primary lymphedema (Marshall Cavendish Corporation, 2007). This phenomenon is consistent with the aetiology of ASMS which has been identified as gene mutations associated with smooth muscles.

It has also been suggested that defects in the lymphatic system account for the increased urinary tract infections in patients suffering from ASMS. This is because the lymphatic system is responsible for fighting infections in the body. Genetic disorders on the lymphatic smooth muscle cells compromise the immune system leading to the persistence of urinary tract infections. On the other hand, the increased urinary tract infections can be caused by the abnormal contractile events of the bladder, ureter and urethral smooth muscles (Webb, 2003). In general, it is possible that ASMS affects the ability of the lymphatic system to drain excess fluids and fight infections.

The occurrence of left systolic heart failure in ASMS patients suggests that the vascular system is affected by defects associated with ASMS. The contractility of the affected vascular smooth muscles causes increase in blood pressure in arteries and veins. Ordinarily, vascular smooth muscles are responsible for controlling the contractility of blood vessels (Hardin & Vallejo, 2006). Evidence shows that abnormal contractions of the vascular smooth muscles may lead to pathology such as ischemia, hypertension and infarction. It is also possible that the rigidity condition in the coronary artery limits blood flow to the left heart muscle leading to left systolic heart failure, more or less the same as the case with coronary artery disease. Therefore, the left systolic heart failure in ASMS suggests that the presence of abnormal contractions in the vascular smooth muscles is due to the smooth muscle gene mutation.

## Conclusion

In conclusion, this essay has demonstrated that ASMS exhibits the same pathophysiology as most contractile smooth muscle disorders which impair the function of organs and tissues with smooth muscles. From a clinical perspective, the main symptoms of ASMS; lymphedema, cyanosis and increased urinary tract infections, suggest the impairment of airway, lymphatic and vascular smooth muscles.

## References

Berridge, M. (2008). Smooth Muscle Cell Calcium Activation Mechanisms. *The Journal of Physiology, 586*(pt21), 5047-5061.

Hardin, C. & Vallejo, J. (2006).Caveolinsin Vascular Smooth Muscle: Form Organizing Function. *Cardiovasc Res, 69*(4), 808-815.

Marshall Cavendish Corporation (2007). *Diseases and Disorders, Volume 2.* Singapore, Singapore: Marshall Cavendish.

Martin, L. (2013). *Cyanosis and the Clinical Assessment of Hypoxemia.* Retrieved from http://emedicine.medscape.com/article/303533-overview#showall

Webb, R. (2003). Smooth Muscle Contraction and Relaxation. *Advances in Physiology Education, 27*, 201-206.

# YOUR KNOWLEDGE HAS VALUE

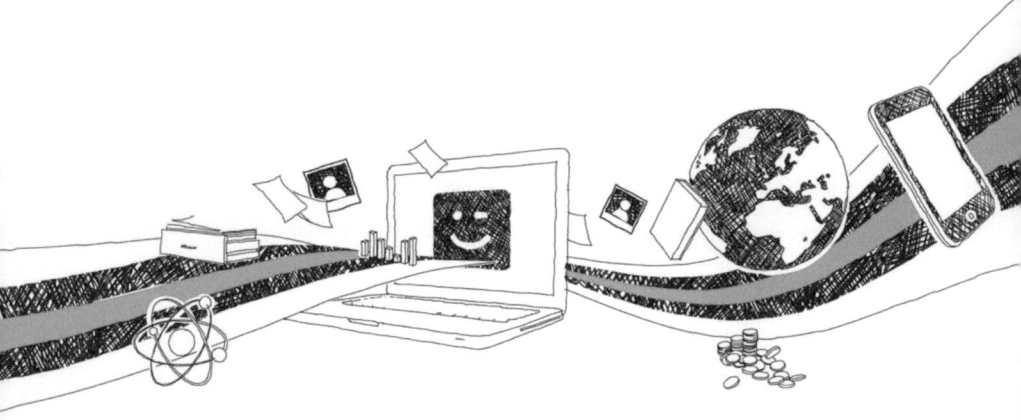

- We will publish your bachelor's and master's thesis, essays and papers

- Your own eBook and book - sold worldwide in all relevant shops

- Earn money with each sale

Upload your text at www.GRIN.com and publish for free

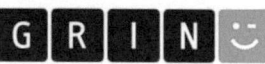